LIVE WHOLE, HEALTHY, AND FREE!
An Inspiring Guide to Living in the Moment

By Jenny King

©2020

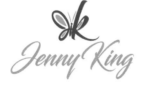

For more information visit: www.jennjennthefriend.com

Cover Design: Primo Design Shop

ISBN 978-1-7355976-1-4 (paperback)

Library of Congress Cataloging-In-Publication Data has been applied for.

Contents

HEY THERE MY FRIEND

I don't take it lightly that you've chosen to read this book, and my heart is filled with gratitude for you. You may be in a place of darkness right now and feeling as though you're at the end of your rope. Trust me, I've been there before too. Or maybe you're doing just fine, and only looking for a little encouragement. Either way, I guarantee there is something in this guide for you.

Before we dive in, may I take just a moment to share one of my truths? I used to live in my head. In fact, I never lived in the moment because I was too busy living in my head. I was so insecure and had the lowest self-esteem imaginable. So self-conscience and self-loathing. The self-list could go on and on for days. I was so empty, broken, and ashamed. I could be in a room full of people and feel so invisible, almost hoping not to be noticed by anyone. I always rehearsed negative thoughts in my head. Over and over again, I'd tell myself that I didn't matter. I rehearsed that negativity so much to the point those negative thoughts became my talk and reality. I didn't like who I was and if I'm completely honest, I didn't *know* who I was. I saw others appearing to live fulfilled lives that flowed from a deeper understanding of themselves, and I wanted to experience life in that way too. I couldn't take living life seeded in negative thinking any longer, and I decided to do something about it.

About 12 years ago I embarked upon an incredible journey of what I like to call whole-self-discovery. And I'm so excited to share the experiences and lessons that I've learned over the years with you. Please hear me when I say there is no magic button here. It took lots of self-work and years of figuring it all out. But I will say what has kept me along the way - the very center of my journey from the beginning has been the Lord Jesus Christ. So, if you're reading this book and struggling with living in your head (just like I did) and you never live in the moment, please know there is hope for us! Start exactly where I did. Start by seeking the Lord Jesus Christ. Seek direction in Him! Find your identity in Him, and I assure you that everything else will fall into place.

Now let's jump right into this guide to living in the moment. May God show us how to Live Whole, Healthy, and Free!

– *Jenny*

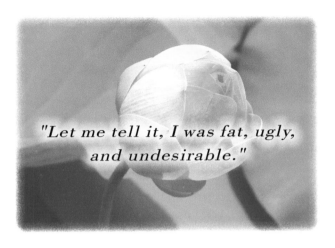

"Let me tell it, I was fat, ugly, and undesirable."

INTRODUCTION

KNOW WHO YOU ARE

I grew up the youngest of two in a loving household with both my parents. We had a musical family, and from an early age I loved the creative arts. Mostly everything I enjoyed doing as a child I still enjoy doing now. Singing, writing, dancing, teaching, cooking, shopping, performing, posing for the camera, oh and of course, eating. I enjoyed eating and boy did I eat a lot growing up. Food was my safety net. I found comfort in food and food found comfort in me. Some of my fondest memories growing up involved food and some of my darkest memories do too. I was always a chubby little girl and I carried the weight all the way into my adulthood. Fast forward to 2008 when my whole-self-discovery journey began. I was fed up with life as I knew it and decided to pack my small apartment at the time and move about four hours away from all my friends and family to a small town where I knew not one soul. I wanted to take a few years to grow into myself. This was one of the scariest but best decisions I made in life, and I can't imagine who I would be today had I not taken that leap of faith 12 years ago.

Despite all the great things I accomplished as a young adult, in my early 30's I reached the lowest point I had ever been in life. I remember it just like it was yesterday. After four years of living in that small town, I was in desperate need of yet another change of scenery. And so, I decided to move back to my home city. I was making just over $30,000 working as an administrative assistant. And I hated where I was in life professionally. Now, there is absolutely nothing wrong with admin work, but I desired so much more for myself, and I knew I was capable of much more. I was depressed and too embarrassed to admit to anyone that my career as a secretary led me to the ladies' room to cry for an hour every day during my lunch break. I had tons of debt and was scraping to get by, living check to check trying to undo the damage I had done living well beyond my means for so many years prior. To top it all off I hated how I looked. Let me tell it, I was fat, ugly, and undesirable. I felt stuck and it seemed to me like everyone else's – and I mean *everyone* else's – situation in life was so much better than mine. But we know that wasn't the case at all.

I struggled with comparing myself to others. I wanted Susie's seemingly happy marriage, Jackie's doting children, Stacy's perfect job, and Mary's beautiful home. I coveted Samantha's hair and skin, Tara's personality, and Judy's great looks. I was so busy looking at everybody else, I couldn't see my own unique and valuable assets. One of the very first lessons I learned on my whole-self-discovery journey was that although comparison is a natural tendency (just like any other emotion) it ultimately is a choice to do it. Comparison can be a very tough habit to break, but if you want to experience the fullness that life has to offer, it is a habit that must be broken. I had to realize that if I wanted to really discover true happiness, I had to acknowledge that comparison was (and still is at times) a huge joy-stealer for me. And the negative effects of it was the root cause of so many broken areas in my life.

One of the most crippling and broken areas in my life was my appearance. My weight! As I said, I struggled with my weight for my entire life. In fact, I don't remember a time when I wasn't overweight. Like so many, I've lost weight over the years only to gain it all back again. Each time losing a bit of confidence in my ability to keep the weight off for good. I seriously started my adult weight loss journey back in 2011, this time doing it for myself. On my own, through exercise and changing my eating habits, I trimmed down seven sizes smaller by 2014. And as I am sure you guessed it, by 2018, after celebrating that win just four years prior, I found myself struggling to keep the weight off yet again. I never publicly acknowledged the weight gain at that time because I honestly didn't realize it until it was too late.

Through life's highs and lows I had packed on more and more of those shed pounds, and by 2018 I was on the verge of tipping the scale at a number not too far from where I started previously in 2011. Needless to say, I was so embarrassed and frustrated. In 2018 I shifted my focus and got even more serious about my whole-self-discovery journey. It's in that shift I began to realize this broken area in my life – the weight – was a direct connection to my self-esteem (how I viewed myself...how I perceived my own self-worth and value). You know if you don't truly value something you will not take care of it. And in this case the "it" was me!

I had to learn to redirect my self-deprecating thoughts and bad habits. I turned that negative behavior into positive daily deposits instead, and I learned to do it because I really and truly cared about Jenny. I mean *really* valued myself. This changed behavior led me to a deeper exploration of who I was. I began to seek a deeper understanding of life and what it meant to live in the moment. Before

I started my journey of whole-self-discovery, I didn't feel alive. It felt as though days were passing me by, and I had no clue how I fit into the mix. I wanted to know what it was like to live in the moment, to intentionally be present and take each minute as a gift – a precious opportunity in time for growth and development. Although over the past several years my amazing journey of whole-self-discovery has gotten extremely difficult at times, the path undoubtedly has led me to true happiness. Or what I like to affectionately call whole-happiness, that is happiness from the inside-out. Being whole-happy is a healing process that fosters transformation. And along the way you learn so much about who you are. Knowing who you are is your superpower. When you find that place of certainty within yourself, nothing and no one can shake that foundation.

Has your story been shaped by brokenness? Are you having a tough time shaking heartache and disappointment? Have you healed from past hurt, but looking for a little positive reinforcement to keep moving in the right direction? Well, if any of that resonates with you, then stick around for more and commit to starting your own personal journey of whole-self-discovery today!

PART I

THE WHOLISTIC SYSTEM

The purpose of our journey
is to restore ourselves to wholeness.
— Debbie Ford

CHAPTER ONE

ENHANCE YOUR LIFE

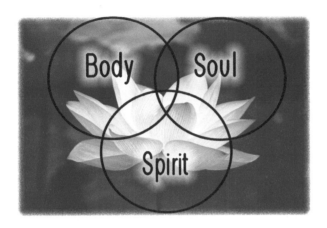

Before we go any further, I want to let you in on a little secret… You are already whole. We are born whole, but life experiences, comparison, poor self-esteem, and other debilitating factors keep us from walking in our wholeness. If you think about it before you plant a seed into the ground, the seed is already the desired outcome it is intended to be. Proper nourishment and cultivation are what determines that seed's potential, growth rate, and destiny. Acknowledging the fact that we are already whole is the first step to wholeness. And recognizing we are a tripartite being is the next.

Tripartite means *wholistically* we are made up of spirit, soul, and body. And to enhance our lives, we must nurture and take into consideration our whole-self – Spirit. Soul. Body. Our spirits are connected to the heart of who we are, from which we receive direction. Deep within our souls, which encompass the mind, will, emotions, and conscience, we find empowerment. And our bodies enable us to create wealth. As a tripartite being, enhancing your life requires continuous development of the spirit, soul, and body, which will ultimately bring *wholistic* wealth. But more on that later…

By 2019 I had found my stride in my weight loss pursuit. I was committed to exercising, eating better, and loving the process. The only problem was that I wasn't seeing much difference on the scale. When you've struggled with weight your entire life like me and start a new fitness regimen, the scale can wreck your self-esteem. I've now come to grips with the fact that fitness cannot just be about weight loss! Instead of obsessing over the number I see on the scale, I have learned to celebrate my non-scale victories as well.

I've learned to embrace my successes as a tripartite being. There are spiritual wins, triumphs that feed my soul, and of course, improvements to my physical body along the way – all worth celebrating. And each of those deserves applause: looking better in my clothes, having more energy, getting stronger – and I mean literally stronger, sleeping better and recognizing the need to properly manage stress, becoming more flexible and able-bodied to jog a little longer and sprint a little faster are all motivating wins (no matter how big or small) that must be celebrated just as much as any progress on the scale.

Now, my outlook on fitness is more about making it a habit to ensure I get a regular dose of endorphins each week, which helps my mental health and overall mood. I also focus on handling emotional eating much better, and that, in turn, helps me to stay on track. Most importantly I've gained the confidence to keep progressing! When I focused solely on a physical weight loss journey (my body), I was taking a fragmented approach to being whole, healthy, and free. I've since shifted my thinking as a result of my whole-self-discovery journey and *wholistically* speaking I am enjoying the celebration of every small victory along the way – Spirit. Soul. Body.

CHAPTER TWO

CULTIVATE THE EIGHT ESSENTIAL ELEMENTS OF YOU

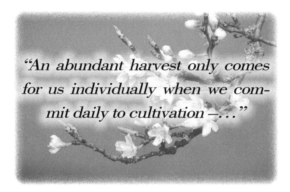

"An abundant harvest only comes for us individually when we commit daily to cultivation —…"

Once you've committed to a lifetime of personal growth and development as a tripartite being – spirit, soul, and body, the next step in your whole-self-discovery journey requires an understanding that we are even more complex than our spirit, soul, and body. In fact, beyond a tripartite identity, there are Eight Essential Elements of You! That's right! Eight Essential Elements of You, and if you're not cultivating each of these areas in your life, you're not taking a *wholistic* approach to your personal growth and development. In *The Wholistic System™*, I've outlined my proven approach to *wholistic* growth and development. Following *The Wholistic System* is how I've managed to get unstuck in life and heal from brokenness.

I used to feel as though I didn't have everything I needed to become all that I wanted to be in life. But on my whole-self-discovery journey, I've realized the exact opposite is true. Just like a plant, our innate abilities and gifts need water, good nutrients, sunlight, the right temperature, space, and time to grow. And just like plants, our visions and aspirations have to be cultivated. Heck! *We* have to be cultivated! Cultivation is the act of caring for something. And abundant harvest only comes for us individually when we commit daily to cultivation – the process of developing ourselves and living intentionally. To walk fully in all that you are, I firmly believe that you must be in the practice or make a habit of cultivating these Eight Essential Elements of You.

1. Mental

Your mental health is extremely important because it impacts how you interact with the world around you. It shapes your coping abilities to handle stress, and ultimately it directs the choices you make in life.

2. Emotional

Emotional intelligence is critical because it requires a deep level of self-awareness. If you can successfully learn how to manage your own emotions, it will enable you to live a more fulfilled life.

3. Relational

People need people and your relational well-being allows you to create a strong support system.

4. Financial

Financial literacy helps you make wise decisions in life. Gaining an appreciation for different perspectives on budgeting, saving, investing, credit, and debt management will give you a leg up. The more you develop this essential element of you, the better.

5. Spiritual

Increasing your knowledge and understanding of spirituality strengthens your connection to your higher power. For me, that means complete reliance on the Lord Jesus Christ and seeking Him for direction and guidance in life.

6. Personal

Personal development encompasses so many things – from talents to potential, to dreams, and aspirations. Continuous development of this essential element is the key driver behind getting unstuck in life whenever you're feeling stagnant.

7. Physical

Physical activity improves your overall health. Learning to embrace the importance of staying active reduces health risks and provides other benefits like heightened self-esteem, mood-enhancement, mental clarity, and aids in better quality sleep.

8. Professional

Good business skills enhance your employability and entre-preneurial mindset. Committing yourself to lifelong learning will set you apart from the pack.

So, what's the point of it all?...

To enhance your life, you must Cultivate the Eight Essential Elements of You! Simultaneously!

And starting out, I highly recommend setting what I like to call a whole-self goal in each essential element group to work towards monthly.

1. Mental
2. Emotional
3. Relational
4. Financial
5. Spiritual
6. Personal
7. Physical
8. Professional

8 Essential Elements of You

NOW THAT WE'VE COVERED *THE WHOLISTIC SYSTEM*, HERE'S MY #WHOLESELFIECHALLENGE TO YOU...

If you're done with negative thinking and you're ready to start cultivating the Eight Essential Elements of You, join my Circle of Friends and take the #WholeSelfieChallenge. All you need to do is:

1. Take a pic of yourself and share on your Instagram and social feeds
2. Include the following text in your caption "I'm enhancing my life with *The Wholistic System!*"
3. Be sure to use the hashtags #WholeSelfieChallenge, #LiveWholeHealthyFree, and #jennjennthefriend
4. Tag me @jennjennthefriend to make sure we don't miss your post

And that's it!

Want to enhance your life? Cultivate the Eight Essential Elements of You!

> **Grab your copy of *The Wholistic System*™ Monthly Tracker and Daily Journal today! This planner will help you track progress on your whole-self-discovery journey.**

PART II

HEALTHINESS IS THE KEY TO WHOLISTIC WEALTH

Life can be challenging at times. I mean, come on, if we're really being honest, life can be downright painful. Over the years, I developed a poor coping mechanism of pushing down all my negative experiences, especially when it came to my issue with weight. Each time, locking my true self further and further away. I recognized early on this was a problem and I set out to undo the damage that had been done. You know the old saying, "Find Yourself!?" Well, I used to think it was a complete joke. That is until I started my own whole-self-discovery journey. I wanted to remove all of those layers that I had built up over the years and get back to my true self.

I've now grown to appreciate the importance of not only knowing who you are but also learned the importance in finding yourself. And that takes diligence and perseverance to uncover. When you finally reach that point of finding yourself on your whole-self-discovery journey, you will unlock the magic that dwells within you. It feels like discovering a pot of gold. Simply put, the way to finding yourself comes through a diligent pursuit of healthiness, and that will lead you to *wholistic* wealth.

If there was one piece of advice that I could share with you, from one friend to another, I'd say never – and I mean *never* – stop striving to be a healthier version of yourself. Never stop striving to unlock your magic and discover that pot of gold. Because a healthy you will have great perspective and fortitude to navigate through life no matter what comes. On my whole-self-discovery journey, I've learned that pursuing healthiness means getting in touch with your true self, which is even more valuable than currency. Keep reading to uncover my Seven Successful Secrets to Healthiness and *Wholistic* Wealth!

CHAPTER THREE

CRACK THE CODE

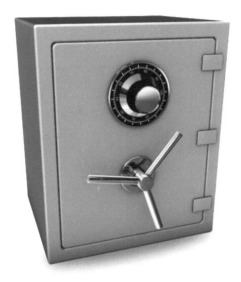

1

SILENCE THE NOISE AND DEFINE SUCCESS FOR YOURSELF.

You must clear out what everyone else is saying and determine what matters most to you.

JOURNAL WITH JENN

Take a moment to connect with your thoughts and feelings. Write down what success is to and looks like for you.

Be still with your thoughts and feelings. Review, reflect, and investigate your journal entry. See your whole-self as you are destined to be regarding defining success for yourself. List one word or draw an image that represents what you envision.

Create your own in-the-moment mantra as it relates to your definition of success by filling in the blank below:

In this moment I (example: am, commit to, feel...)

_____.

2

DEVELOP YOUR BEST SELF-CARE ROUTINE.

Find ways to refuel yourself daily.

JOURNAL WITH JENN

Take a moment to connect with your thoughts and feelings. Write down what self-care means to and looks like for you.

Be still with your thoughts and feelings. Review, reflect, and investigate your journal entry. See your whole-self as you are destined to be regarding self-care. List one word or draw an image that represents what you envision.

Create your own in-the-moment mantra as it relates to your best self-care routine by filling in the blank below:

In this moment I (example: am, commit to, feel...)

_____.

3

IDENTIFY YOUR SUPPORT SYSTEM.

None of us has the strength to do life alone. Invest time and energy into building meaningful relationships.

Journal with Jenn

Take a moment to connect with your thoughts and feelings. Write down what characteristics you need in your support system and who those individuals are. It's ok if you don't know them yet. Now is a great opportunity to put yourself out there and network to find and build those relationships.

Be still with your thoughts and feelings. Review, reflect, and investigate your journal entry. See your whole-self as you are destined to be regarding your support system. List one word or draw an image that represents what you envision.

Create your own in-the-moment mantra as it relates to your support system by filling in the blank below:

In this moment I (example: am, commit to, feel...)

_____.

CHAPTER FOUR

UNLOCK YOUR AUTHENTIC SELF

4

Don't neglect the inner-self work.

Dive deep into your past traumas, figure out your triggers, heal from those past hurts, and allow yourself to transform.

JOURNAL WITH JENN

Take a moment to connect with your thoughts and feelings. Write down all your past traumas and triggers that come to mind. The purpose is to seek healing and self-understanding.

Be still with your thoughts and feelings. Review, reflect, and investigate your journal entry. See your whole-self as you are destined to be regarding healing from your past hurts. List one word or draw an image that represents what you envision.

Create your own in-the-moment mantra as it relates to your inner-self work by filling in the blank below:

In this moment I (example: am, commit to, feel...)

_____.

5

FOCUS ON SELF-LOVE.

Confidence starts from within! Learn to value yourself and stop settling for less than you deserve in life.

JOURNAL WITH JENN

Take a moment to connect with your thoughts and feelings. Write down what self-love means to and looks like for you.

Be still with your thoughts and feelings. Review, reflect, and investigate your journal entry. See your whole-self as you are destined to be regarding self-love. List one word or draw an image that represents what you envision.

Create your own in-the-moment mantra as it relates to your self-love experience by filling in the blank below:

In this moment I (example: am, commit to, feel...)

_____.

6

FACE YOUR FEARS.

If you never try, you'll never know what it feels like on the other side. Be brave and believe in yourself.

JOURNAL WITH JENN

Take a moment to connect with your thoughts and feelings. Write down what scares you most and the fears that are holding you back.

Be still with your thoughts and feelings. Review, reflect, and in-vestigate your journal entry. See your whole-self as you are destined to be regarding facing your fears. List one word or draw an image that represents what you envision.

Create your own in-the-moment mantra as it relates to your vic-tories over fear by filling in the blank below:

In this moment I (example: am, commit to, feel...)

_____.

CHAPTER FIVE

GET BACK TO A HEALTHY YOU

7

THINK. DO. BE.
WASH, RINSE, AND REPEAT!

Think your way into *Doing* what naturally forces you into *Being* Whole, Healthy, and Free! If that doesn't excite you then I don't know what will. Simply put, you are the key to unlocking your authentic self. You are what you think, and you become what you put into practice daily.

I'll say it once more for good measure... *Think* your way into *Doing* what naturally forces you into *Being* Whole, Healthy, and Free!

Journal with Jenn

Take a moment to connect with your thoughts and feelings. Write down what the affirmation *Think. Do. Be.* means to you.

Be still with your thoughts and feelings. Review, reflect, and investigate your journal entry. See your whole-self as you are destined to be regarding being whole, healthy, and free. List one word or draw an image that represents what you envision.

Create your own in-the-moment mantra as it relates to being whole, healthy, and free by filling in the blank below:

In this moment I (example: am, commit to, feel...)

_____.

In summary, a diligent pursuit of healthiness will lead to *wholistic* wealth. Crack the code, unlock your authentic self, and get back to a healthy you with my Seven Successful Secrets to Healthiness and *Wholistic* Wealth!

1. Silence the noise and define success for yourself.

2. Develop your best self-care routine.

3. Identify your support system.

4. Don't neglect the inner self-work.

5. Focus on self-love.

6. Face your fears.

7. Think. Do. Be.
Wash, rinse, and repeat!

Now take each of your in-the-moment mantras, post them around your living and workspaces, and speak positivity over your whole-self daily!

PART III

A LIVING-IN-THE-MOMENT MENTALITY WILL KEEP YOU FREE

I know but one freedom
and that is the freedom of the mind.
— Antoine de Saint-Exupery

CHAPTER SIX

DON'T HOLD YOURSELF HOSTAGE

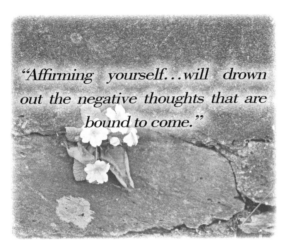

"Affirming yourself...will drown out the negative thoughts that are bound to come."

Like I mentioned before, I've struggled with weight my entire life. In fact, I can't remember ever being a "normal" size. Ever! The only memory I have of me as a smaller size is captured in one childhood picture. I loved posing for the camera as a child, and I have one special picture of me as a kid before I became chubby and fat. I pull that out from time to time to reflect upon. That picture reminds me of the freedom I once had. It was a time before I became so insecure. It was before I developed the lowest self-esteem imaginable. That one image reminds me of the time before I became so self-conscience and self-loathing. We'll call the little girl in that image the whole, healthy, and free Jenny.

She was so full of life, love, and carefree. Weight wasn't an issue for her and thoughts of herself were not dictated by societal pressures. She was herself and showed up every day with love and light simply as herself. My primary goal throughout my entire whole-self-discovery journey has been to get back to who I was in that picture from my childhood. It is not necessarily that I want to get back to a small size but I want the wholeness, healthiness, and freedom that little Jenny exuded in that image.

One of the more recent lessons I've learned on my whole-self-discovery journey is that a living-in-the-moment mentality will keep you free. On this journey it is so important to figure out what is holding you hostage. For many, that bondage starts in our minds. Limiting beliefs can stifle you and will keep you from experiencing all that life has to offer. The barriers that I created in my mind held me hostage for so many years and manifested through emotional eating, weight gain, and a poor self-image.

My whole-self-discovery journey forced me to face my triggers. I had to really dig deep and determine what would set me off on food binges. I then had to find other ways to deal with those stressors and emotions. I also had to remove stimulants from my surroundings like stop buying the junk food that I so easily depended on for comfort. That shift in viewpoint taught me to make better food choices while developing healthier life habits overall. I had to find the balance between tracking my progress with weight loss and not obsessing over the number on the scale. But I also learned along the journey that it is crucial to not neglect checking progress on the scale because the number on the scale is an important factor. It's just not the *only* factor in measuring success. Finally, I've learned that probably the most critical part of all is to be kind to yourself. If the mental picture you have of yourself is not rooted in kindness, then it's likely you are holding yourself hostage.

Ultimately, we hold ourselves hostage in our minds, in the way we think about ourselves and view situations. That is why I believe in daily affirmations. Affirming yourself – be it with scripture, positive quotes, motivational recordings, or mantras developed on your own – will drown out the negative thoughts that are bound to come.

We just can't let the negativity overtake us. Remain in control and unshackled by choosing to think and speak positivity over yourself – daily. And that is why I charged you to develop your own in-the-moment mantras earlier in this book.

If you get in the habit of speaking those affirmations daily, it will help you develop a living-in-the-moment mentality. After you've done the inner self-work required throughout your whole-self-discovery journey in order to unlock your true, authentic self, you will want to remain free. To accomplish that, which is no small feat, you have to make the choice every day to maintain a living-in-the-moment mentality. Even when life feels awful and gets disappointing, it is in how we choose to respond that makes all the difference. And a positive outlook will yield positive results of freedom.

CONCLUSION

LIVE WHOLE, HEALTHY, AND FREE!

You've made it this far in the book which means I haven't bored you. I've shared some of my darkest moments with you and also revealed how I managed to overcome them. It's so easy to want to rush through life and to want to race to the finish line. But I want to stress to you that your whole-self-discovery journey does not have an end point. As tripartite beings, we are constantly evolving, especially when we are committed to a lifetime of personal growth and development.

Now, let's reflect on what I've covered in this guide. First things first, you have to stop comparing your life and situations to others. If you are not happy with the way things are, do something about it. Change any bad habits that might be holding you back and cease the negative thinking that is feeding that poor self-talk. Focus on wholeness that is spirit, soul, and body while committing to continuously cultivating the Eight Essential Elements of You. Get back to who you are with my Seven Successful Secrets to Healthiness and *Wholistic* Wealth. Allow your true self to not be held captive by your mind. Maintain perspective in all things. And now, most importantly, live in the moment. It's not enough to just be whole, healthy, and free. No! I want you to *live* whole, healthy, and free. I want you to know what it is like to live in the moment, to really be present, and take each moment in as a gift - a precious opportunity in time for growth and development.

Above all, my whole-self-discovery journey has taught me to strive to live by the saying "seize the moment" and now I firmly believe every moment we have is a gift to be cherished and experienced fully. Living in the moment is living with intention. And living intentionally requires a wholehearted connection to *The Wholistic System*. Get out of your head and be present. Being present takes courage to fully experience every pain, joy, failure, and success along the way. Your whole-self-discovery journey will be revealing. There will be highs and many lows. At times, the path will get tough and might even seem scary. But I guarantee the road ahead will undoubtedly lead to true happiness. Just as it did for me, your whole-self-discovery journey will lead to whole-happiness. And being whole-happy is a healing process that fosters transformation, meaning, purpose and intentionality.

So, there you have it! This guide was birthed from years of trial and error. And years of tough lessons, tears, pain, joy, and fulfillment have ensued as a result. I'm sharing my story with you because I want to see you walk in all that life has to offer. Do not think for one second that things can change overnight. As tripartite beings, we just are not built that way. Anything worth having is worth the work. And Yes - it takes work to commit to a lifetime of growth and development. Doing the work yields an abundant life and the prerequisite to an abundant life is the pursuit of whole-happiness, that is happiness from the inside-out. Want to know exactly how to live in the moment? Well, the answer lies in this very moment. See your whole-self as you are destined to be and commit to a lifetime of whole-self-discovery.

I'll leave you with this final thought. If there is nothing else the past 12 years on my whole-self-discovery journey has taught me...it's that living in the moment can be summed up into these four simple words – Live Whole, Healthy, and Free!

May God lead you on your whole-self-discovery journey every step of the way!

HOW TO CONNECT WITH JENNY

I hope you enjoyed this guide to living in the moment! If you're looking for comprehensive support then you'll want to check out my free offers, online courses, live events, and personal development products.

Intentional living begins where Wholeness and Productivity meet. Now that you've read this book on wholeness, attend my free webinar, *Master Your Morning*, to start living with intention. Also, look out for more info on my Productivity Resources and join the fun.

To learn more visit jennjennthefriend.com.

Follow me on Instagram and Facebook @jennjennthefriend.

Also, be sure to join *Jenn's Circle of Friends* and subscribe to my email list at jennjennthefriend.com.

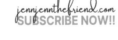

SUBSCRIBE NOW!!

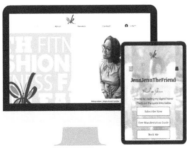

TAKE THE #WHOLESELFIECHALLENGE NOW!
ALL YOU NEED TO DO IS:

1. Take a pic of yourself and share on your Instagram and social feeds.

2. Include the following text in your caption: "I'm enhancing my life with *The Wholistic System!*"

3. Be sure to use the hashtags: #WholeSelfieChallenge, #LiveWholeHealthyFree, and #jennjennthefriend

4. Tag me @jennjennthefriend to make sure we don't miss your post.

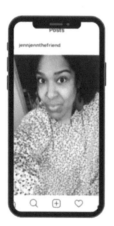

I'm enhancing my life with
The Wholistic System!
#WholeSelfieChallenge
#LiveWholeHealthyFree
#jennjennthefriend

NEXT STEPS

WOW!

Take a deep breath in and out...

You made it to the end.

I hope this guide has inspired you to never lose sight of your whole-self-discovery journey.

As a bonus offer, I am including three journal prompts below to help with developing your living-in-the-moment mentality.

1. What parts of your life are most distracting?

2. Reflect on specific distractions that keep you from living-in-the-moment. List them and explain why each is a distraction.

3. Spend time today being fully present and engaged. Remove all external and internal distractions. Reflect on how you spent your day, and how your time living-in-the-moment made you feel.

DON'T FORGET TO GRAB A COPY OF *THE WHOLISTIC SYSTEM* MONTHLY TRACKER AND DAILY JOURNAL. THIS PLANNER WILL HELP YOU TRACK PROGRESS ON YOUR WHOLE-SELF-DISCOVERY JOURNEY.

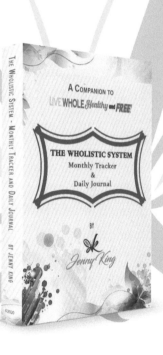

Praise from Followers:

"It has been a blessing on my life to have reconnected with Jenny and to benefit from her powerful messages of self-love and faith. I love how she keeps it all the way real and I can relate to so much, if not all, of her content. I absolutely love seeing how she has grown into this dynamic woman who continues to allow God to use her in ways that honor Him and the gifts He's placed in her that benefits anyone who tunes into her messages."
-Nicole K. Harris

"I find Jenny's blog posts/topics really resonate with me and my audience. It is so important while we are adjusting to our 2020 new normal and the separation of personal and physical connections because of COVID-19 that we have a powerful voice of positivity that builds individuals up and inspires and lifts up, instead of tearing them down. JennJennTheFriend is truly a friend to all."
-Corey Blackwell

"JennJennTheFriend goes above and beyond to live up to her name. The moment I see a new story/post from her, I'm eager to know what the topic is going to be about. Jenn is a great motivator. She will have you engaged and wanting to do more with her, and in your personal life as she gives some advice to reaching personal goals."
-Samona Ewing

"I appreciate the honesty and transparency in the content that Jenny shares. Not only is it inspiring. It also motivates me on my journey as well."
-Brian D.

Image Credits:

Image on page 7 by Jo Spargo from Pixabay.

Image on page 13 by Hong Zhang from Pixabay.

Image on page 15 by Uschi Dugulin from Pixabay.

Safe photo pg. 23, This Photo by Unknown Author is licensed under CC BY-NC, August 2020.

Safe photo pg. 45, This Photo by Unknown Author is licensed under CC BY-SA, August 2020.

Image on page 47 by Manfred Richter from Pixabay.

Section break art by AnnaliseArt from Pixabay.

CPSIA information can be obtained
at www.ICGtesting.com
Printed in the USA
LVHW070345030221
678221LV00001B/6